TAKING ACTION TO REDUCE TOBACCO USE

National Cancer Policy Board

Institute of Medicine and
Commission on Life Sciences, National Research Council

NATIONAL ACADEMY PRESS
Washington, D.C. 1998

NATIONAL ACADEMY PRESS • 2101 Constitution Avenue, N.W. • Washington, D.C. 20418

NOTICE: The project that is the subject of this report was approved by the Governing Board of the National Research Council, whose members are drawn from the councils of the National Academy of Sciences, the National Academy of Engineering, and the Institute of Medicine. The members of the National Cancer Policy Board, which is responsible for the report, were chosen for their special competences and with regard for appropriate balance.

This report has been reviewed by individuals chosen for their diverse perspectives and technical expertise, in accordance with procedures approved by the NRC's Report Review Committee. The purpose of this independent review is to provide candid and critical comments that will assist the authors as well as the NRC and IOM in making the published report as sound as possible and to ensure that the report meets institutional standards for objectivity and evidence. The content of the review comments and draft manuscript remain confidential to protect the integrity of the deliberative process. We wish to thank the following individuals for their participation in the review of this report: Harvey Fineberg, *Coordinator*, Harvard University; Virginia Weldon, *Monitor*, Monsanto Corporation; Neal Benowitz, University of California, San Francisco; Frank Chaloupka, University of Illinois, Chicago; Jack Henningfield, Pinney Associates and Johns Hopkins University; Thomas Houston, American Medical Association; Michael Pertschuk, The Advocacy Institute; and Kenneth Warner, The University of Michigan.

While the individuals listed above have provided many constructive comments and suggestions, responsibility for the final content of this report rests solely with the National Cancer Policy Board, the NRC and IOM.

The Institute of Medicine was chartered in 1970 by the National Academy of Sciences to enlist distinguished members of the appropriate professions in the examination of policy matters pertaining to the health of the public. In this, the Institute acts under both the Academy's 1863 congressional charter responsibility to be an adviser to the federal government and its own initiative in identifying issues of medical care, research, and education. Dr. Kenneth I. Shine is president of the Institute of Medicine.

The National Research Council was organized by the National Academy of Sciences in 1916 to associate the broad community of science and technology with the Academy's purposes of furthering knowledge and advising the federal government. Functioning in accordance with general policies determined by the Academy, the Council has become the principal operating agency of both the National Academy of Sciences and the National Academy of Engineering in providing services to the government, the public, and the scientific and engineering communities. The Council is administered jointly by both Academies and the Institute of Medicine. Dr. Bruce M. Alberts and Dr. William A. Wulf are chairman and vice chairman, respectively, of the National Research Council.

This study was supported through funding provided by the National Cancer Institute (Contract No. NO2-CO-71024), Centers for Disease Control and Prevention, American Cancer Society, Amgen, and Abbott. The views presented in this report are those of the National Cancer Policy Board and are not necessarily those of the funding organizations.

International Standard Book No. 0-309-06038-9

Additional copies of this report are available for sale from the National Academy Press, Box 285, 2101 Constitution Avenue, N.W., Washington, D.C. Call (800) 624-6242 or (202) 334-3313 (in the Washington metropolitan area), or visit the NAP's on-line bookstore at **http://www. nap.edu.**

This report is available on-line at **http://www.nap.edu/.** For more information about the Institute of Medicine or the the National Cancer Policy Board, visit the IOM's home page at **http://www2.nas.edu/iom** or the NCPB's home page at **http://www2.nas.edu/ cancerbd.**

Copyright 1998 by the National Academy of Sciences. All rights reserved.

Printed in the United States of America

NATIONAL CANCER POLICY BOARD

PETER HOWLEY[*,†] (*Chair*), George Fabyan Professor and Chair, Department of Pathology, Harvard Medical School
JOSEPH SIMONE (*Vice-Chair*), Medical Director, Huntsman Cancer Foundation and Institute, University of Utah
JOHN BAILAR,[*] Chair, Department of Health Studies, University of Chicago
NORMAN DANIELS, Professor of Philosophy, Tufts University
JOSEPH DAVIE,[*] Vice President, Department of Research, Biogen, Inc., Cambridge, Mass.
ROBERT DAY, President and Director, Fred Hutchinson Cancer Research Center, Seattle
KATHLEEN FOLEY,[*] Chief of Pain Service, Department of Neurology, Memorial Sloan-Kettering Cancer Center, New York City
BERTHA FORD, Coordinator, Cancer Clinical Trials, The Arthur G. James Cancer Hospital and Research Institute, Columbus, Ohio
ELLEN GRITZ, Professor and Chair, Department of Behavioral Sciences, University of Texas M.D. Anderson Cancer Center, Houston
ELIZABETH HART, President and CEO, Hart International, Dallas
JOHN LASZLO, Independent Consultant, Atlanta
WILLIAM McGUIRE,[*] Chief Executive Officer, United HealthCare Corporation, Minnetonka, Minn.
DANIEL NATHANS,[†] Senior Investigator, Howard Hughes Medical Institute, Bethesda, Md., and Professor of Molecular Biology and Genetics, Johns Hopkins University School of Medicine
SANDRA NICHOLS, Director, Arkansas Department of Health, Little Rock
DIANA PETITTI, Director, Research and Evaluation, Kaiser Permanente Medical Care Program, Pasadena, Calif.
AMELIE RAMIREZ, Associate Professor, Department of Medicine, Baylor College of Medicine
WILLIAM ROPER,[*] Dean, University of North Carolina School of Public Health, Chapel Hill
JOHN SEFFRIN, Chief Executive Officer, The American Cancer Society, Atlanta
JANE SISK, Professor, Columbia University School of Public Health
ELLEN STOVALL, Executive Director, National Coalition for Cancer Survivorship, Silver Spring, Md.
FRANCES VISCO, President, National Breast Cancer Coalition, Philadelphia
ROBERT YOUNG, President, Fox Chase Cancer Center, Philadelphia

---

[*] Member, Institute of Medicine.
[†] Member, National Academy of Sciences.

Special Contributor

RICHARD J. BONNIE, John S. Battle Professor of Law, and Director, Institute of Law, Psychiatry, and Public Policy, University of Virginia School of Law

Study Staff

ROBERT MULLAN COOK-DEEGAN, Director
STACEY PATMORE, Senior Project Assistant
KATHLEEN McCORMALLY, Research Assistant and Summer Intern
CATHARYN LIVERMAN, Program Officer

IOM Staff

MICHAEL STOTO, Senior Staff Officer, Division of Health Promotion and Disease Prevention
JANE DURCH, Program Officer, Division of Health Promotion and Disease Prevention
CLAUDIA CARL, Reports and Information Office
MICHAEL EDINGTON, Reports and Information Office

Contents and Recommendations

BACKGROUND 2

RAISE PRICES TO REDUCE USE 4
The price of tobacco products must be increased substantially, 4
Failure to achieve targeted reductions in youth consumption should result in further manufacturer-specific penalties, 5

STRENGTHEN FEDERAL REGULATION 7
FDA must continue to regulate tobacco products, and the U.S. Congress must strengthen and clarify FDA's role, 7

SUPPORT STATE AND LOCAL TOBACCO CONTROL EFFORTS 9
The federal government must support state and local infrastructure for tobacco control, 10
Congress must repeal the federal preemption of state and local regulation of advertising and promotion, 11

MONITOR PERFORMANCE IN RELATION TO PUBLIC HEALTH GOALS 11
The federal government must establish a system for performance monitoring in collaboration with other levels of government and private organizations, 11

HELP CURRENT USERS QUIT 18
Effective smoking cessation interventions, as identified by the AHCPR guidelines, should be widely disseminated and incorporated into the standard of practice, 18

Government health programs and private insurance and health plans should cover treatment programs for tobacco dependence, 18

Treatment programs for tobacco dependence should be incorporated into quality of care measures, "report cards" on health plans, and public health performance monitoring, 19

Programs and norms outside the medical care system must also support prevention, cessation, and harm reduction, 19

SUPPORT RESEARCH 20

Federal research agencies must increase their commitment to research on tobacco control, 20

The U.S. Congress and Public Health Service agencies should intensify research on tobacco-related diseases, 22

FDA and NIH should mount research programs to improve future regulation, 23

The federal government must support research to clarify the feasibility, risks, and benefits of "harm reduction" strategies, 24

FACILITATE INTERNATIONAL TOBACCO CONTROL 25

The United States must promote, participate in, and contribute funds to the building of a capacity for evaluating and monitoring international tobacco control efforts, 26

The United States should refrain from implementing trade policies that undermine foreign tobacco control efforts, 27

The United States can study and learn from effective foreign tobacco control policies, 29

SUMMARY 30

REFERENCES AND NOTES 31

TAKING ACTION TO REDUCE TOBACCO USE

Taking Action to Reduce Tobacco Use

The nation needs a strategy to reduce the death and disability caused by use of tobacco products. That strategy may develop out of a renascent public debate about tobacco control policies that has intensified over the past three years. When the Institute of Medicine (IOM) released its 1994 report, *Growing Up Tobacco Free,*[1] prospects for federal action were highly uncertain. That same year, the surgeon general's report was also focused on youth tobacco use.[2] Prospects for tobacco control grew brighter when the Food and Drug Administration (FDA) asserted jurisdiction over tobacco products, with strong presidential support, state attorneys general brought suit against tobacco firms on a new legal basis, and class-action lawsuits became more palpable threats to the financial future of private tobacco firms. Media coverage of these events and revelations of hitherto secret files and depositions from former tobacco firm employees has been intense. These and other developments have resulted in a vigorous national debate about tobacco control among the various groups with a stake in tobacco policy—tobacco firms, state attorneys general and health officials, public health groups, tobacco growers, tobacco control advocates, and others. Attention now focuses on the U.S. Congress and the executive branch, which are seriously considering federal legislation.

Although public debate has intensified, tobacco use among youths has escalated. Smoking rates among youths have increased for four years in succession (1993–1996), as measured by the largest national survey, the University of Michigan's "Monitoring the Future" project.[3] Today's tobacco use will become tomorrow's health statistics. As a four-decade longitudinal study of smoking in British physicians concludes, "about half of all regular cigarette smokers will eventually be killed by their habit."[4] New users will become addicted to nicotine, followed years later by a sharply increased incidence of tobacco-related diseases. Cancer, cardiovascular disease, and lung disorders cause most tobacco-related deaths, although tobacco use is associated with many other medical conditions. Among the 419,000 Americans who died from smoking in 1990, for example,

151,000 died of cancer. The increased numbers of deaths among women are particularly alarming. Since 1987, more women have died each year of lung cancer than breast cancer. An American Cancer Society graph illustrates the dramatic rise in the rate of lung cancer among women, which follows the rise in women's smoking that began several decades earlier.[5]

There are only three basic ways to reduce the death toll: to prevent the initiation of tobacco use, to get current users to quit, and to reduce exposure to tobacco toxins. The vast majority of those who use tobacco start doing so in childhood or youth, so prevention efforts must focus there. Individuals of all ages can quit using tobacco, and the cessation of tobacco use is associated with immediate economic and health benefits from reduced cardiovascular disease[6] and long-term reductions in the likelihood of developing cancer.[7] Reduced exposure to tobacco toxins has followed from bans in public places.

Preventing the initiation of tobacco use among children and youths remains the preeminent long-term goal, but cessation of tobacco use by individuals in all age groups is also essential. The projection that 10 million people will die of tobacco-related illness in the year 2030 is mainly based on the number of current users.[8] This enormous health toll will thus drop only if current users quit and are not replaced by other users, and if tobacco exposure is reduced. The worldwide health consequences also clearly indicate that national tobacco control policies must look beyond national borders.

At its first two meetings in the spring of 1997, the National Cancer Policy Board identified tobacco control as a priority, and tobacco control was the subject of its initial policy statements. The board organized a workshop on July 15, 1997, in Washington, D.C., and summarized its views in a July 18, 1997, letter to Secretary of Health and Human Services Donna Shalala, the president's Domestic Policy Advisor Bruce Reed, and members of the U.S. Congress. This white paper builds on those efforts, addressing (a) price increases, (b) federal regulation, (c) state and local tobacco control programs, (d) performance monitoring, (e) cessation programs, (f) research, and (g) international health impacts.

BACKGROUND

Even as the IOM Committee on Preventing Nicotine Addiction in Children and Youths was completing its work in 1994, FDA was beginning an investigation that culminated in the precedent-setting regulation of tobacco products. This effort began with a petition to FDA Commissioner David Kessler in February 1994 from the Coalition on Smoking OR Health and culminated in an assertion of FDA's jurisdiction over tobacco products under the Food, Drug, and Cosmetics Act. Following an extensive FDA investigation, in August 1995 President Bill Clinton announced his intention to assert FDA jurisdiction over tobacco products as nicotine-delivery devices. (A more complete chronology of events leading to the FDA action is available on-line at: **http://www.os.dhhs.gov/news/press/1996pres/960823f.html.**)

Most states have also brought suit against tobacco firms to recoup state funds expended on health care for those suffering from tobacco-related diseases. In May 1994,

Michael Moore, the attorney general of Mississippi, filed the first such lawsuit. In August 1994, Minnesota Attorney General Hubert H. Humphrey III filed a similar suit. Since then 38 more states and many city and county governments have joined Mississippi and Minnesota in filing suits against tobacco manufacturers. In March 1997, the Liggett Group, Inc., reached a settlement with the attorneys general of five states and, a few days later, with the plaintiffs in one of the class-action suits. This agreement acknowledged that nicotine is addictive and that marketing has been directed at youths. Liggett also agreed to make public previously secret industry documents.

On June 20, 1997, the attorneys general of 40 states announced an agreement (hereafter "the settlement") with five additional tobacco firms, which among them account for more than 95 percent of tobacco sales in the United States. The settlement would entail payments of up to $368.5 billion over 25 years. The settlement proposed FDA regulation, marketing and promotion restrictions, some antitrust exemptions for tobacco firms, and liability limits with escrow funds for class-action, individual, and state suits. On July 3, 1997, Mississippi reached its own settlement of more than $3 billion, but this will be superseded by the congressionally ratified settlement if it comes to fruition. On August 25, 1997, Florida reached an $11.3 billion settlement that would likewise be superseded by federal legislation, except that a $150 million pilot tobacco control pilot program will continue with or without federal settlement. A three-phase Texas Medicaid suit was scheduled to begin in October 1997, but this was delayed until January 1998 due to the judge's illness. The suit brought by Minnesota is scheduled to go to trial in January 1998.

In addition to the actions of the state attorneys general and FDA, dozens of individual and class-action lawsuits have been filed against tobacco firms. Suits have also been filed in several countries in Europe, Latin America, Asia, and Africa. On October 9, 1997, a class-action suit brought by flight attendants was settled out of court, creating a $300 million fund. Those funds "shall be used solely to establish a Foundation [the Norma Broin Foundation, named for the flight attendant who initiated the suit] whose purpose will be to sponsor scientific research with respect to the early detection and cure of diseases associated with cigarette smoking."

The various lawsuits have forced to the surface documents related to the tobacco industry. In December 1997, the House Committee on Commerce issued subpoenas for over 800 documents identified in connection with the Minnesota state suit, and made them publicly available. In addition to the courtroom drama, industry whistleblowers have publicly disclosed previously secret documents and practices, and the 1996 U.S. presidential campaign featured a lively debate about tobacco control.

Despite a mounting debate, consensus about the details of national tobacco control policy is not complete. Public health advocates differ sharply about whether a national settlement is desirable at all, let alone about the terms of such a settlement. With expressions of support for legislation from both the president and the leaders in the U.S. Congress, however, the debate has shifted from theory into the political arena. The findings and recommendations of this report are directly pertinent to the policy decisions now under active consideration, including but by no means restricted to legislation related to the settlement.

Several bills have been introduced in late 1997, and several other bills are being actively drafted with the expectation they will be introduced early in 1998.[9] Federal tobacco control legislation will touch upon the jurisdictions of diverse committees in both houses of Congress. Judiciary committees may address the liability and antitrust provisions, health committees (the Senate Labor and Human Resources Committee and the House Commerce Committee) may address the public health and research provisions, agriculture committees may address the implications for tobacco growers, commerce committees may address the marketing and advertising of tobacco products, education committees may address the components dealing with public education, and tax policy committees (the Senate Finance Committee and the House Ways and Means Committee) may address the revenue implications. These committees held many hearings in the last four months of 1997, and congressional attention is expected to continue in the final session of the 105th Congress in 1998. In addition to legislation growing out of debate about a settlement, Congress will be making decisions about appropriations for enforcement of the FDA rule, federal research and tobacco control programs, and oversight and conduct of U.S. contributions to international tobacco control. This report is intended to inform the debate about federal tobacco control policies in Congress, in the executive branch, and among other stakeholders. The remainder of this white paper addresses recommendations to policymakers, organized according to methods for reducing tobacco use.

RAISE PRICES TO REDUCE USE

The price of tobacco products must be increased substantially.

Raising the prices of tobacco products is a proven way of reducing tobacco use in the short and medium terms. Price hikes both encourage cessation and thwart initiation. Higher prices have the added benefit of reducing use among people not yet addicted to nicotine, including young people, whose level of tobacco consumption may be more sensitive to price.[10] The impact and simplicity of price hikes were the main reasons that the 1994 IOM report's first recommendation was a $2 per pack cigarette tax increase (and an equivalent increase for other tobacco products). The recommended increment had three goals: to achieve the desired reduction in demand, to attain rough parity with the most effective tobacco control programs in other countries,[11] and to avoid creating a black market. A significant price increase was also recommended recently in the report of a committee chaired by former Surgeon General C. Everett Koop and former FDA Commissioner David A. Kessler. The National Cancer Policy Board believes that a $2 price increment remains the single most effective way of reducing overall tobacco consumption. Such a price increase should also have the desired disproportionately greater impact on preventing the initiation of tobacco use among young people.

There are many ways to raise prices. A federal excise tax is simple and direct and would create a revenue stream that could be used for research and tobacco control measures. An excise tax increment has the virtue of being collected through existing structures appropriated with other federal funds. The main argument against a federal excise tax increment is political pragmatism—any tax increase is suspect, and a tobacco excise tax hike of this magnitude has never been passed by Congress. The federal tobacco excise tax was increased by 15 cents (to be phased in) in the Balanced Budget Act of 1997, but this is far less than recommended and encountered stiff opposition. There are also concerns about any new taxes and about the regressive nature of taxes that fall on current tobacco users.

The settlement proposes that the tobacco industry make payments into a fund and stipulates certain broad principles for spending those funds, subject to allocation by a board. The industry payments are an alternative mechanism to a tax and would similarly raise prices. This process leaves many unanswered questions and relies on institutions that must be created de novo. Negotiation of the allocation process could well prove to be complicated, with many interested parties staking contending claims, because tobacco firms, tobacco farmers, health researchers, tobacco control activists, state governments, state and federal health programs, international tobacco control efforts, and others all have a stake.

The proposed settlement has the virtue of ensuring that some funds are used to promote public health, to advertise the health dangers of tobacco use, to carry out research, and to support other tobacco control measures. This link between tobacco revenues and tobacco control measures has been implemented in state efforts, such as those in Arizona, California, Massachusetts, and Oregon. This linkage mitigates the unpopularity of tax increases. The mixed uses of funds derived from tobacco revenues for health programs or education as well as tobacco control, however, has proven to be troublesome, particularly in the first years of the California program.[12] Use of tobacco excise tax funds has also been contentious elsewhere, but a fraction of the funds from state excise taxes has successfully been devoted to tobacco control efforts in Arizona and Massachusetts. Tobacco tax collection has never been linked to tobacco control efforts at the federal level, and partially for this reason, federal tobacco control initiatives have been anemic. The State of California, for example, spends more on tobacco control than the entire federal government.[13] Ensuring that some tobacco revenues go to tobacco control could be achieved by legislative set-asides in combination with tax increases, without the need to create a new mechanism for obtaining payments from industry or for the allocation of a new pool of funds. Regardless of whether existing processes are used to allocate funds or new ones are created, the process should be insulated to the degree possible from raw politics. Funds allocated for research, for example, would most fruitfully be directed through peer-reviewed channels at the National Institutes of Health (NIH). In program areas in which such peer-review mechanisms do not exist, they should be created.

Failure to achieve targeted reductions in youth consumption should result in further manufacturer-specific penalties.

Goals for reducing tobacco use among youths and adults are specified in *Healthy People 2000*,[14] and the settlement proposes that the rate of smoking among youths be reduced by 60 percent over a decade. The proposed settlement incorporates some penalty payments if the rate of smoking among youths is not reduced, but the penalties are capped and there are provisions for rebates to be given to firms on the basis of good faith efforts. Price increases and other measures incorporated into the settlement would surely result in improvements to public health compared to the status quo, but they may fall short of achieving the specified goals.

The payments in the proposed settlement will likely not raise tobacco prices sufficiently to achieve demand reduction goals through price increases alone. Analysts have reached widely differing conclusions about the impact of the proposed settlement on tobacco consumption among youths. Despite wide agreement that higher prices reduce the level of tobacco consumption,[15] the magnitude of the effect depends not only on price but also on what other measures are taken and how effective they are. A drop in youth consumption is likely, but its magnitude cannot be predicted with precision. A 10 percent price increase could reduce consumption by as little as 4 percent, according to some estimates, or by as much as 12 or 13 percent, according to others.[16] Tobacco use may also be influenced, moreover, by restrictions on access to tobacco by youths, advertising and promotion, and other measures.

The Federal Trade Commission recently released a report on the economic implications of the proposed settlement. It projects an ultimate price increase in the range of 62 cents per pack and estimates that the actual present value of the proposed settlement is in the neighborhood of $100 billion to $120 billion (as opposed to the face value of $368.5 billion, with the lower amount resulting from inflation, demand reduction, and other factors). Jeffrey Harris of the Massachusetts Institute of Technology, in a report for the American Cancer Society, estimates the net current value of the settlement to be $195 billion.[17] An analysis by researchers at the University of California at San Francisco finds that the funding would be insufficient to recoup Medicaid costs for the treatment of tobacco-related illnesses, let alone to cover the desired tobacco control expenses. An industry analysis differs with these assessments. It projects an eventual price increase of 83 cents per pack under the settlement, with a greater reduction in the level of tobacco consumption and sharply lower profits.[18] A response from the Federal Trade Commission notes the out-year price projections in the industry analysis are not adjusted for inflation. FTC also challenges the assertions about effects on profits.[19]

The board cannot resolve the uncertainty over how much tobacco prices will increase, the effect of price increases on consumption, or the additive effect of price on other tobacco control measures. The board believes, however, that the desired health goals should dictate tax rates (or settlement payments) rather than the reverse. Fixing the tax rate or payment amount in advance, with no provisions for adjustments later in light of data about levels of consumption and the initiation of tobacco use among youths, invites failure to achieve the public health goals. If tobacco consumption and initiation do not recede, taxes on tobacco products should be increased to further reduce demand. Any tax increases or penalty payments should be indexed to inflation, so the effects on consumption and the revenues to support tobacco control and other goals are not eroded over time. A system of public health monitoring, as suggested below, is needed to guide pricing interventions, such as taxes or penalties under any settlement legislation.

The American Cancer Society urges elimination of the penalty caps and rebates in the settlement. The American Society of Clinical Oncology suggests a "fail-safe mechanism," with excise tax increases triggered by failure to attain youth tobacco-use targets. The American Medical Association lists several provisions to redesign the penalties if youth consumption goals are not met, including a provision that "payments should be assessed against each individual company based on reductions in underage use achieved by that company. They should not be assessed on the basis of collective industry responsibility."[20]

Incentives to reduce youth tobacco use will be most powerful if penalties for failure to achieve goals fall hardest on those firms making brands attractive to underage users. If youth tobacco initiation goals are not met, financial penalties should be targeted to manufacturers, based on brands used disproportionately by youths.[21] The board recommends that payments triggered by failure to reach public health goals should be structured into any federal legislation. A flat excise tax, based on the weight of the tobacco content, does not provide this incentive because each firm retains the incentive to lure young smokers, thus building a future market, yet penalties are distributed evenly across all tobacco products.

Even states with active tobacco control campaigns have seen increases in tobacco use among young people in recent years, although at rates lower than the national average.[22] These states, however, have not seen tax increases of the magnitude now contemplated. Effects of Alaska's tax increase to $1 per pack that went into effect in October, Hawaii's two-step increase scheduled to reach $1 per pack in June, and New Jersey's recently doubled tobacco tax (to $0.80 per pack) should generate data soon, but those increases are still only half the increment recommended by the board. If an initial tax increase (or settlement payment) of $2 per pack (and the equivalent for other tobacco products) fails to reduce use among youths to target levels, payments from firms making brands popular among should be increased to induce further price increases.

STRENGTHEN FEDERAL REGULATION

FDA must continue to regulate tobacco products, and the U.S. Congress must strengthen and clarify FDA's role.

In 1994, IOM recommended that the U.S. Congress enact a comprehensive regulatory statute delegating to an appropriate agency "the necessary authority to regulate tobacco products, for the dual purpose of discouraging consumption and reducing the morbidity and mortality associated with use of tobacco products." The report recommended that the agency be authorized to regulate the design and constituents of tobacco products, and specifically discussed the possibility of setting and gradually reducing ceilings on the nicotine content of tobacco products. FDA was noted as one agency that could exercise the recommended authority. The board believes subsequent events have demonstrated that FDA is the logical lead for tobacco regulation.

A year after the release of the IOM report, FDA formally proposed to regulate tobacco products using its existing authority under the Food, Drug, and Cosmetics Act. The agency enacted final regulations in 1996. FDA's Tobacco Rule regulates the advertising and marketing of tobacco products and the distribution of these products to minors, but it does not address the design and constituents of tobacco products. If the courts uphold FDA's assertion of jurisdiction over tobacco products, the agency will have broad authority to move beyond the current rule to regulate the design and content of tobacco products as well.

The courts may or may not ratify FDA's jurisdiction over tobacco products. On April 25, 1997, Federal District Court Judge William Osteen upheld FDA's assertion of jurisdiction, but he struck down certain provisions. That ruling is now on appeal to the Fourth U.S. Circuit Court of Appeals. The case is likely to be reviewed by the U.S. Supreme Court. This process might take several years, and the outcome cannot be predicted with confidence. Moreover, even if FDA's jurisdiction over tobacco products is upheld, its scope of authority under existing law is likely to remain uncertain. Although the district court upheld the agency's regulation of distribution to minors, for example, it held that the act did not empower the agency to regulate the advertising and marketing of tobacco products.

In light of the indeterminacy of FDA's existing legal authority—and the imperfect fit between the unique challenges of tobacco control and the regulatory regime set up under the Food, Drug, and Cosmetics Act—national policy would be clearer if Congress were to enact a specific regulatory statute for tobacco products, as recommended in the 1994 IOM report. Congressional action would avoid wasteful and unnecessary litigation and would establish a strong political and legal foundation for future regulatory initiatives. Congress must also appropriate funding to FDA commensurate with its authority. The settlement proposes that FDA regulatory authority expand beyond the terms of the settlement only if FDA can establish that such measures will not create a black market. Proving that something that already exists in many countries will not occur here is an unreasonable burden and would hamstring FDA before it is clear whether the current regulations and new measures proposed in the settlement will achieve their goals. Moreover, it is also premature to foreclose any regulatory authority until there has been full public disclosure of information about the health risks and addictive potential of tobacco products. Congress, FDA, and the public need time to review information currently held by private firms and their attorneys before making irrevocable choices about regulatory strategy and regulatory authority.

The need for congressional action regarding FDA's efforts to restrict tobacco advertising, promotion, and marketing is particularly urgent. Most FDA provisions restricting advertising and promotion are in abeyance pending the federal appeals court decision, and there will be further delay if the case goes to the U.S. Supreme Court. Advertising and promotion constraints may not have dramatic short-term effects, but they are integral parts of all successful tobacco control efforts in states and foreign countries and must be part of any long-term U.S. national tobacco control program. The 1994 IOM report recommended comprehensive regulation of advertising and promotion that tends to encourage young people to use tobacco products. Recommendations included restricting advertisements to text-only format and bans on promotional campaigns attractive to youths. Although the FDA regulation implements many of these ideas, the federal district court ruled that the agency does not have the statutory authority to regulate tobacco advertising and marketing, without even reaching the industry's argument that these regulations violate the First Amendment to the Constitution. Even if the agency's jurisdiction to regulate youth access to tobacco products is upheld, FDA's scope of authority over advertising and marketing will be in litigation for many years. Congressional action to implement IOM's 1994 recommendations would expedite the nation's tobacco control agenda by many years.

Public debate regarding the desirability of the proposed settlement has highlighted the thorny issues of regulatory design. Is the best course, for example, to follow the logic of progressively reducing nicotine exposure? What criteria should govern the regulatory agency's decision to initiate, implement, or terminate such a strategy? In what way should the agency take into account the emergence of a black market for illicit tobacco products? Some leaders of the public health community have criticized the criteria set forth in the proposed settlement on the grounds that they would unduly constrain FDA authority compared with the authority now conferred by the Food, Drug, and Cosmetics Act. Others have pointed out that the courts may not uphold FDA's assertion of jurisdiction over tobacco products. They have also argued that the criteria outlined in the proposed settlement provide a suitable starting point for congressional deliberation and the drafting of legislation.

The board cannot resolve this debate, and it does not intend to try to do so. The board does, however, urge Congress and the executive branch to take the necessary steps to ensure that possible strategies for regulating the design and constituents of tobacco products are given careful and systematic study. FDA's authority must be broad enough to allow it to protect the public health on the basis of scientific knowledge as it accumulates. Under some possible regulatory initiatives, an adequate scientific foundation already exists. Studies clearly indicate, for example, that smokers adapt to cigarettes labeled and machine-tested as low in nicotine by inhaling more often or more deeply.[23] Informational requirements regarding tar and nicotine yield could be changed in light of actual human exposures from tobacco products, for example cigarette labeling that takes account of smoking behavior and not just machine-determined yield. On some issues, such as nicotine reduction, regulation must await new research or access to the results of studies now available only to private tobacco firms. In other areas, new information should be available in the coming years. Proposals for long-term nicotine maintenance using FDA-approved nicotine products will require further research. Studies of antidepressant and antiopiate drugs to enhance cessation are also promising, but not enough studies have been completed to reach firm conclusions. Yet the success of treating tobacco dependence and consumer acceptance may well indicate whether regulation of nicotine in tobacco products is a viable option. As another example, some states are experimenting with higher age limits for legal tobacco sales. Such experiments should be encouraged, because the results can help guide national policy. Some regulatory decisions, however, cannot be made until entirely new studies are designed and carried out, and their results are analyzed.

SUPPORT STATE AND LOCAL TOBACCO CONTROL EFFORTS

Current attention to tobacco control follows many years of innovative work at the state and local levels initiated by governments and private organizations. States such as California and Massachusetts have mounted effective public education campaigns, supported research, encouraged local nonsmoking ordinances, restricted some forms of advertising and promotion, and implemented other tobacco control measures. These efforts are funded by increases in state excise taxes on tobacco products. Such increases have also become law in Arizona, Hawaii, and Oregon. As noted previously, Alaska and Hawaii have each raised the state excise tax on cigarettes to $1.00, with Washington and New Jersey approaching that level. Maine, Wisconsin, and Utah are mounting new tobacco control programs. Much of the action in tobacco control has been and will continue to occur at the state, county, and community levels.

The federal government must support state and local infrastructure for tobacco control.

Many increases in nonfederal excise taxes and restrictions on advertising, promotion, and levels of exposure to environmental tobacco smoke depend on the actions of state and local governments. Bans on smoking in public places and in workplaces not only reduce environmental tobacco exposure to nonsmokers, but have also proven to be powerful interventions to enhance cessation and to reduce the dose exposure among smokers. The vast majority of progress on this front has taken place at the state and local levels. Counteradvertising and public education have also been largely state and local efforts, although they would likely be more effective if implemented nationally. All of these are elements of tobacco control efforts and complement federal measures. Success at the federal, state, and local levels has depended in part on funding not only government efforts, but also nongovernment organizations that can hold federal, state, and local governments to account. This pattern of funding should be designed into future tobacco control programs. For now, attention is focused on the terms of the proposed national settlement. If the settlement is translated into legislation, it should provide funding for state and local tobacco control efforts. If no settlement results, however, state and local efforts will nonetheless likely remain the bulwark of tobacco control.

Most federal support comes from the ASSIST program of the National Cancer Institute (NCI) and the IMPACT program of the Centers for Disease Control and Prevention (CDC). California and Massachusetts fund the largest state programs. States that are part of the ASSIST program spend less, but more per state and with more intensive interventions than IMPACT states. In effect, for the past few years, states have engaged in a dose-response test of tobacco control. Evidence from that experiment was presented at the July 1997 IOM workshop; it showed that the program impact roughly parallels the intensity (dose) of tobacco control efforts. California and Massachusetts have the largest programs and greater decrements in tobacco consumption than ASSIST states, which in aggregate show a 7–10 percent greater reduction in consumption than IMPACT states (i.e., all others). These programs are reviewed in the 1994 IOM report, which recommended that federal support for state efforts be increased to the level of ASSIST in all states, with the increase in funding that would entail. This is, in essence, a recommendation to implement ASSIST as a universal program, based on its demonstration in one third of the states. The new evidence reinforces the 1994 recommendation. It is time to apply the lessons of ASSIST nationwide.

Implementing the transition has several implications. First, it is important that the program content of ASSIST be carried forward as it is expanded. This includes retaining program elements as well as drawing on the expertise of those at NCI, in the ASSIST states, and in the nongovernmental organizations that have made it a success. Second, it entails a differentiation in function. As a universal program, it is logical to shift responsibility to the nation's public health agency, CDC. This would entail a significant scaling-up of current efforts. Yet expansion of the CDC effort should not detract from further progress. Tobacco control efforts will be expanding in Alaska, Arizona, Hawaii, Maine, Oregon, Utah, Wisconsin, and other states. The ASSIST program has shown that a more intense intervention produces results, but it does not clearly show which elements are most powerful, and ASSIST states could not test counteradvertising, public education, or other interventions at the level possible in California and Massachusetts. An expanded commitment to tobacco control increases the importance of knowing which interventions matter most, requiring demonstrations at sufficient dose and duration to enable credible evaluation. That is, many questions remain for research, high-intensity demonstrations, and rigorous program evaluation. This is no time to retrench from research or to stop testing even larger-scale demonstrations. The goal for the next decade should be to achieve tobacco control rivaling that in California and Massachusetts, through the use of a combination of state, local, and federal funds and any payments resulting from a national settlement, and to improve the programs in all states through research, demonstrations, and program evaluation.

Congress must repeal the federal preemption of state and local regulation of advertising and promotion.

The most successful efforts to curb tobacco use have grown from mobilization at the state and community levels and have entailed collaborations among private health organizations and federal, state, and local governments. Federal legislation currently prohibits state and local governments from regulating any form of advertising and promotional activities based on smoking and health, even if the activity occurs exclusively within states' jurisdictional borders. The opportunity for innovation at the state and local levels would be enhanced if this federal impediment were removed, as recommended in the 1994 IOM report.

MONITOR PERFORMANCE IN RELATION TO PUBLIC HEALTH GOALS

The federal government must establish a system for performance monitoring in collaboration with other levels of government and private organizations.

No matter what the final settlements about federal policy prove to be, federal action alone is insufficient to achieve tobacco control. Regardless of which tobacco control measures are put in place, both local and national capacities must be in place to translate goals into actions, to measure progress, and to provide feedback for subsequent policy decisions. The massive national effort that went into *Healthy People 2000* is a good place to start a discussion of public health goals.[24] *Healthy People 2000* devoted a chapter to tobacco use, specifying national goals on a timetable; the goals for reducing tobacco use among youths, however, are further from achievement than they were even a few years ago.

A recent IOM report, *Improving Health in the Community*,[25] proposes ways of bridging the gap between national goals and community action and identifying specific organizations or groups at the community level accountable for making progress toward those goals. The general approach discussed in the report is embodied in the Community Health Improvement Process (CHIP). CHIP applies the tools used to monitor performance. To promote the achievement of health improvement goals, the approach entails (a) specifying goals, (b) developing a strategy to achieve them, (c) identifying and implementing local interventions that can be monitored by quantitative indicators, and then (d) collecting and assessing performance data for the specific accountable entities at the community level to evaluate the effectiveness of the intervention strategy and the contributions of the specific accountable entities in the community. The accountable entities will vary among communities, as will the relative priorities of the goals and the resources available to attain those goals.

The CHIP approach might be adapted for use at the national level as well. National health improvement goals might be translated into intervention strategies that federal agencies and a variety of national organizations might be expected to act on and for which performance indicators might be developed and monitored. Such activities at the national level might help shape related efforts at the state and local levels. The approach is described at greater length, with its theoretical underpinning and with specific consideration of tobacco control issues, in a separate background paper prepared for the board by Michael Stoto and Jane Durch of IOM (available on-line at **http://www2.nas.edu/cancerbd/226e.html**).

Three elements are central to the IOM CHIP model: (1) a broad view of health as a product of the interaction of many factors; (2) recognition that protecting and improving health is a shared responsibility of many entities, each of which needs to be accountable for its activities; and (3) a performance monitoring framework, in which sets of actionable measures are tied to specific entities that can help to ensure the necessary accountability. Accountability is a concern because responsibility diffused among many entities can easily be ignored or abandoned. This approach also points to the importance of interventions that focus not only on individuals but also on collective actions such as the adoption of policies to limit smoking in workplaces or restaurants or the enforcement of laws prohibiting the sale of tobacco products to persons under age 18. In extending the CHIP concept to the national level, there may be opportunities to focus on interventions that target communities and organizations rather than individuals.

A well-chosen set of performance measures could help to reinforce a balanced national and local tobacco control effort. The CHIP approach calls for the use of sets of indicators to make meaningful assessments of overall performance because health issues have many dimensions and can be addressed by various sectors. These sets of indicators should cover critical features of a health improvement effort. They should, however, remain selective; too many details can obscure the broader picture. Indicators must be carefully selected to provide insight into the progress that has been achieved. For an issue such as tobacco control, for which changes in health outcomes such as a reduction in lung cancer deaths will not be observable in the near term, the set of indicators should balance measures of shorter-term gains (e.g., reductions in smoking prevalence or sales of tobacco products to minors) and more fundamental longer-term changes in health (e.g., reductions in the incidence of lung cancer or lung cancer mortality). The approach is perhaps best explained by way of an illustration, showing some possible national and local performance measures (see table, page 14).

The objectives in *Healthy People 2000* are an essential reference point for developing performance measures at the national or the community level. The proposed FDA regulations that mandate restrictions on the sale of tobacco products to youths will be an appropriate focus for performance monitoring, even if other FDA provisions are not implemented. The proposed settlement also stipulates specific goals for reductions in the rate of smoking among youths that could guide the development of performance indicators. Likewise, the recommendations made by the Koop-Kessler Advisory Committee on Tobacco and Public Health suggest a variety of performance measures that might be used to monitor progress.

Without an overall monitoring plan, there is real danger of focusing on one or a few measures to the exclusion of others. The proposed settlement, for example, stipulates extra payments from tobacco firms if smoking measures for youths do not improve. The trigger is the level of daily smoking reported in surveys of youths conducted by the University of Michigan. This measure, part of the larger Monitoring the Future study, could change, even without real changes in the rate of initiation.[26] Initiation of tobacco use often begins well before high school and often progresses over two to three years. A more sensitive indicator, such as whether tobacco products were used in the previous 30 days, could also be used (with differential weight) earlier in the process to monitor tobacco use among those in younger age groups. These measures hinge on how students, excluding those not attending school, recall and report their smoking behavior. These measures are useful, but they should be balanced with other independent measures, such as smoking rates among those in the youngest age categories of the National Health Interview Survey, as suggested in the proposed performance measures (see tables). Otherwise, the high stakes create strong incentives to "game" a single indicator without changing the underlying behavior. Self-report measures are notoriously subject to interpretation and recall bias. The point is not that levels of smoking among youths reported in one survey or another are inaccurate or misleading—all measures are limited in one way or another—but rather that caution must be taken against relying on a single measure to monitor performance.

Some fraction of any additional revenues that become available should be devoted to getting better measures more frequently and to making them publicly available. Credible brand-specific penalties or tax increases as recommended above, for example, would require firm data the government could rely on when assessing the payments or taxes. At present the public health monitoring process is slow and coarse compared to the data available to individual tobacco firms.

Reducing tobacco use will require a broader set of measures, reflecting not only the initiation of tobacco use among youths but also the cessation of tobacco use among individuals in all age groups and the attainment of policy objectives. It will also require assessment at the community level as well as in national measures. The performance measures in the table mentioned above are merely first rough cuts to illustrate the possibilities of performance monitoring. The specific measures and objectives can surely be refined, but any long-term strategy for tobacco control must confront the problem: Broader and more robust ways of promoting and monitoring progress and evaluating the relative success of different interventions in diverse communities are needed.

National and Local Performance Measures to Monitor Tobacco Control Efforts

Issue/National Performance Measure	Stakeholders/ Responsible Entities	Possible Corresponding Community Indicators	Possible Stakeholders/ Responsible Entities
Smoking-related mortality • Number of deaths nationally due to lung cancer, cardiovascular disease, emphysema, chronic bronchitis, respiratory infections; percentage of these deaths attributable to smoking	• National health care organizations, federal government, business, national organizations, general public	• Number of deaths in the community due to lung cancer, cardiovascular disease, emphysema, chronic bronchitis, respiratory infections; percentage of these deaths attributable to smoking	• Health care providers and plans, state and local health agencies, business, community organizations, special health-risk groups, general public
Adult smoking • Percentage of the adult population, ages 18 and older, who smoke regularly		• Percentage of the adult population, ages 18 and older, who smoke regularly	• State and local health agencies, business, community organizations, general public
Initiation of tobacco use • Percentage of 8th, 10th, and 12th graders who have used cigarettes or smokeless tobacco in past 30 days • Percentage of 8th, 10th, and 12th graders who use cigarettes or smokeless tobacco daily • Percentage of those ages 20–24 who smoke regularly • Percentage of males ages 12–24 who use smokeless tobacco regularly	• Federal government, national voluntary organizations, general public		• State and local health agencies, schools, community organizations, general public
Access of children and adolescents to tobacco • Development of national regulations regarding youth access • Implementation of regulations by manufacturers (minimum package size; limits on self-service displays, mail order sales and coupons, free samples)	• Food and Drug Administration (FDA), Congress • Manufacturers	• Effectiveness of local enforcement of laws prohibiting tobacco sales to youths (minimum age, minimum package size; limits on vending machines, self-service displays, free samples)	• State and local health agencies, local government, business, industry, general public

Goal	Responsible parties	Indicators	Responsible parties
Reduce appeal of tobacco to youths	• FDA, Congress • Manufacturers	• Development of national regulations regarding advertising directed at youths • Implementation of regulations by manufacturers (text-only format, sponsorship of events, sales/distribution of nontobacco items) • Implementation of regulations by manufacturers (no billboards near schools and playgrounds) • Extent to which tobacco use prevention is incorporated into school curricula and activities	• Local health agencies, local government, schools
Reduce exposure to environmental tobacco smoke (ETS)	• Federal government, national businesses, national voluntary organizations	• Development of model ETS regulations • Prevalence of ETS regulations in federal government facilities • State and local regulation of smoking in workplaces and enclosed public places • Enforcement of existing ETS regulations	• State and local health agencies, local government, business, industry
Promote cessation of tobacco use	• Federal government, national health care plans, national voluntary organizations, national business organizations	• Federal funding for development and evaluation of smoking cessation programs • Cessation attempts among the adult population, ages 18 and older, who smoke regularly • Availability of smoking cessation programs • Cessation attempts among the adult population, ages 18 and older, who smoke regularly	• Health care providers/plans, business, community organizations, general public
Smoking during pregnancy	• Federal government, national health care plans, national voluntary organizations, national business organizations	• Federal funding for development and evaluation of smoking cessation programs for pregnant women • Cessation among pregnant women who smoke regularly • Availability of smoking cessation programs for pregnant women • Cessation among pregnant women who smoke regularly	• Health care providers/plans, business, community organizations, general public

Continued

National and Local Performance Measures to Monitor Tobacco Control Efforts (*continued*)

Issue/National Performance Measure	Stakeholders/ Responsible Entities	Possible Corresponding Community Indicators	Possible Stakeholders/ Responsible Entities
Health care system efforts to reduce tobacco use • Percentage of smokers whose health care providers ask about smoking, provide cessation counseling, and assist with cessation efforts • Proportion of nonsmoking youths counseled not to begin tobacco use • Percentage of healthcare-plan-covered lives with coverage for tobacco cessation programs • Proportion of health plans or national professional organizations that have adopted policies or recommendations that during appropriate health care visits clinicians should identify patients who use tobacco, provide cessation counseling, and assist in cessation efforts • Proportion of academic health centers that include training in cessation counseling in undergraduate and continuing education curricula for health professionals (including physicians, nurses, dentists, physicians' assistants, etc.)	• Federal government, national health care plans, national voluntary organizations, national business organizations	For each health care plan: • Percentage of smokers whose health care providers ask about smoking, provide cessation counseling, and assist with cessation efforts • Proportion of nonsmoking youths counseled not to begin tobacco use • Percentage of healthcare-plan-covered lives with coverage for tobacco cessation programs	• Health care providers/plans, business, community organizations, general public

Community-based programs to change social norms			
• Federal funding for development and evaluation of community-based programs to change social norms and reduce tobacco use	• Federal government, national businesses, national voluntary organizations	• Existence of community-based antitobacco coalitions • Number of smoking cessation programs available and their use and success rate • Extent to which tobacco use prevention is incorporated into school curricula and activities • Proportion of students who associate physical or psychological harm with and who perceive social disapproval of regular use of tobacco	• State and local health agencies, schools, community organizations, general public
Tobacco excise tax			
• Federal excise tax per pack of cigarettes	• Federal government, manufacturers, smokers, general public	• State excise tax per pack of cigarettes	• State government, manufacturers, smokers, general public

HELP CURRENT USERS QUIT

More than 50 million Americans use tobacco products regularly, including 44 million who smoke cigarettes or cigars or who use spit and snuff tobacco.[27] Approximately 70 percent of smokers express a desire to stop smoking (CDC, 1996). Half attempt to quit each year, but only 2.5 percent succeed (CDC, 1993). At present, approximately 3,000 children and youths start to smoke each day, contributing 1 million new smokers annually (Surgeon General, 1994; IOM, 1994). Even if prevention efforts reduce this figure by 60 percent, the goal stipulated in the settlement each year, the nation will have 400,000 new smokers each year, the majority of whom will become addicted and have difficulty stopping. On top of these compelling public health reasons, there is also a moral reason to intensify cessation efforts: Current tobacco users will be paying the increased prices, and some fraction of that revenue should redound to help them directly.

Dependence on tobacco, including smoking, is a pharmacologically based, behavioral disorder. Treatment is not uniformly integrated into medical practice, and coverage of cessation services is fragmented and incomplete. Addiction to tobacco is a chronic, relapsing disorder; multiple attempts to quit smoking are often required to attain permanent cessation. More than 45 million former smokers in the United States attest to the feasibility of cessation, but the process is difficult. It needs to be made easier, through research and routine integration of cessation services into medical practice.

Effective smoking cessation interventions, as identified by the AHCPR guidelines, should be widely disseminated and incorporated into the standard of practice.

The Agency for Health Care Policy and Research (AHCPR), with cofunding from CDC, has prepared a clinical practice guideline on smoking cessation for primary care physicians and other health professionals. This guideline is based on an exhaustive review of studies performed between 1978 and 1994.[28] The American Medical Association used a grant from the Robert Wood Johnson Foundation to disseminate this guideline to 200,000 doctors and is working with the American Association of Health Plans on the guidelines to be used in managed care organizations. These are welcome steps, but implementing the recommendations of the AHCPR guideline will take time and will require sustained commitment until use of the guideline becomes routine. This requires educating physicians and other health professionals as well as incorporating coverage for cessation programs into insurance and health plans. Moreover, guidelines will need to be updated periodically.

Government health programs and private insurance and health plans should cover treatment programs for tobacco dependence.

The AHCPR guideline notes that successful smoking cessation correlates with the intensity of the cessation regimen. In the short term, cessation is associated with lower rates of cardiovascular disease.[29] In the long term, cancer risks are reduced dramatically, although some genetic damage does appear to be permanent.[30] The Robert Wood Johnson Foundation recently called for proposals to address treatment for tobacco dependence in managed care.[31] The Koop-Kessler report notes that "coverage for tobacco use cessation programs and services should be required under all health insurance, managed care and employee benefit plans, as well as all Federal health financing programs (e.g., Medicare and Medicaid)." The board concurs. Many who quit do so only after repeated attempts, so effective coverage cannot be a one-time benefit but must recognize the cyclical nature of quitting, and health programs must provide coverage for repeat attempts at cessation.

Treatment programs for tobacco dependence should be incorporated into quality of care measures, "report cards" on health plans, and public health performance monitoring.

Assisting smokers with smoking cessation is a powerful intervention for promoting health and reducing dramatically the risk of cancer, heart disease, lung disorders, and other medical conditions. Instruments used to evaluate the quality of health plans and the adequacy of insurance coverage should include an indicator of whether tobacco cessation services are covered. When coverage is included, the effectiveness of the cessation methods needs to be continually measured and reported. This will require ongoing research to improve smoking cessation methods and to assess their cost-effectiveness. The HEDIS measures of health plan quality developed by the National Committee for Quality Analysis, for example, assess whether those enrolled in the plan are advised to quit smoking. Test indicators (provisional measures being evaluated for their usefulness) include how many smokers quit and what fraction of enrollees smoke. These are welcome initial steps, but there is a large gap between rendering advice and affecting quit rates. Access to treatments for tobacco dependence, beyond the general "chemical dependence" measure currently in place, would be a more specific and direct measure. A recent survey of those in health plans asked "Is smoking cessation a covered service in your plan?" and 40 percent of respondents said no; access was higher in staff model health maintenance organizations than in practice associations or network plans.[32]

Adolescent smokers have proven to be more resistant to treatment than adults, and in research trials they have exhibited higher failure rates than adults. This suggests that among research priorities, aspects of treatment for adolescents (motivation, recruitment, retention, adherence, and the long-term effectiveness of behavioral and pharmacological treatments) should rank high. A recently announced NIH program on prevention and cessation of tobacco use among youths should begin to fill this gap.[33]

Programs and norms outside the medical care system must also support prevention, cessation, and harm reduction.

Many tobacco users succeed in quitting without a cessation program and without formal care in the medical system. In recent years, nicotine gum and patches have been approved for sale without prescription (i.e., "over the counter"), and nicotine nasal sprays, lozenges, and aerosols are in the pipeline. Ironically, the market for smoking cessation means that firms making cessation products may apply sophisticated marketing and promotion techniques to entice tobacco users to quit[34] similar to those tobacco firms have used to lure people into taking up tobacco use in the first place.[35] Competition among cessation product manufacturers and service providers also appears to be intensifying. This has the potential to increase public education, encourage a social norm friendly to cessation, and reduce the costs of cessation products and services. The annual Great American Smokeout sponsored by the American Cancer Society is the focus of enhanced media attention and in 1996 incorporated paid public service announcements in tandem with increased advertisements by nontobacco nicotine products. The event was associated with an increase in cessation attempts as measured by surveys and sales of nicotine products.[36]

As more products and services become available, the infrastructure supporting cessation programs will have to grow, and some of this infrastructure will depend on publicly funded health programs at the state and federal levels, in addition to activities in the private sector. With increased attention to cessation however, the quality of cessation programs must be maintained; allowing a proliferation of programs of limited efficacy just because program funding is available would be a waste of resources. C. Tracy Orleans observed that "far and away the greatest need is to do a much better job of disseminating and delivering the treatments we [already] have."[37] Cessation programs must be monitored for their effectiveness as well as participation levels. This will be possible only with continued support of training, monitoring of program quality, and refinement of cost-effectiveness measures.

SUPPORT RESEARCH

Federal research agencies must increase their commitment to research on tobacco control.

The federally funded ASSIST and IMPACT programs have augmented the innovation at the state level noted previously. As more states implement higher intensity tobacco control measures, the value of information to guide those efforts will increase. Any funding derived from new taxes or settlement payments will further increase the need for information to guide tobacco control efforts. Leadership on the research to help guide national tobacco control efforts should come from federal health research agencies. NCI served the nation well by pioneering demonstrations of COMMIT and ASSIST. The National Institute on Drug Abuse (NIDA) has supported important work on addiction, ranging from neuroscience to behavioral and social science. The health toll of tobacco use is as significant for heart and lung disease as it is for cancer. The National Heart, Lung, and Blood Institute has demonstrably improved the nation's health through its National High Blood Pressure Education Program,[38] a major public education program, and its Framingham and MRFIT studies have contributed insights about the health effects of tobacco. It could contribute more of its considerable expertise and resources to the problem of tobacco control.[39]

Two working groups of NCI's Board of Scientific Advisors recently made recommendations to the National Cancer Advisory Board. A report on cancer control observed that:

> Although effective interventions have been developed, their efforts tend to diminish over time as a result of competing messages and lack of booster programs. Few effective interventions are available for youth most at risk, such as those from low-income, less-educated families. . . . Particular attention needs to be given to developing effective interventions for children at early ages, when influence from adults is likely to be most effective. Attention must also be paid to children's social contexts influencing tobacco use, including parents, schools, and communities.[40]

That working group went on to observe the salutary effect of the ASSIST program. A different working group on prevention previously recommended that NCI "Increase the investment in developing effective interventions for prevention and cessation of tobacco use, particularly in populations where tobacco use has remained high, e.g., adolescents, women, and those with less education and income." The working group on prevention differed from the one on cancer control working group about ASSIST, recommending that NCI "Increase the proportion of the tobacco control investment in basic research and in the development of effective interventions, and decrease the investment in large-scale dissemination efforts, e.g., ASSIST."

The board believes that both reports clearly point to a need for an enhanced research effort, including a grants program for social, behavioral, and biological questions pertinent to tobacco control. They also point to a need for large-scale demonstrations and evaluations that will require significant funding and staff effort.[41] The purpose of the ASSIST program was to demonstrate the potential for intervention, and it has done this, becoming the model for nationwide implementation recommended above. Yet a national ASSIST program cannot be an end, but only a beginning. Are workplace and public smoking bans the most effective control measures at the local level? Do youth access restrictions work, and do they reduce youth consumption, or just purchases by minors? Do public education and counteradvertising campaigns have an impact, and is there a "dose" effect? What counteradvertising approaches actually work? Should prevention messages be targeted at youths, or is that counterproductive? These and many other questions needed to help guide future tobacco control efforts cannot be addressed through small research grants alone. They require federal research agencies to commit significant resources to help design and fund high-intensity interventions, to fund rigorous evaluation of federal and state-funded programs, and to disseminate those findings. They will also entail interactions with nongovernmental groups with expertise in social marketing, social science, and community interventions. The resources freed from research budgets by the transfer of ASSIST should be augmented and devoted (a) to fund research grants, (b) to support trials of new preventive and treatment interventions, and (c) to plan and carry out intensive new demonstrations needed to guide national tobacco control efforts.

The U.S. Congress and Public Health Service agencies should intensify research on tobacco-related diseases.

The federal government, through NIH and other Public Health Service agencies, is uniquely capable of sustaining a robust research program on the health consequences of tobacco use as a component of the tobacco control research agenda suggested above. Several of the recommendations in earlier sections implicitly call for research, ranging from research in areas of molecular biology to social science, behavior, and prevention. In a July 31, 1997, statement to the Senate Judiciary Committee, the American Association for Cancer Research urged "Congress to ensure that the resources provided through the tobacco settlement will: (1) markedly increase the cancer research budget of the NCI; (2) underwrite the cost of participation in clinical research trials on tobacco-related cancers that will contribute to curative or preventive new therapies; and (3) supplement, not supplant, current resources provided to the NIH and NCI." The Society for Research on Nicotine and Tobacco similarly noted that "research must be substantially expanded to ensure progress in our ability to curtail the development of nicotine addiction and to effectively treat a broader range of nicotine-addicted people. This includes research ranging from the molecular basis of nicotine's action to genetic influences on the vulnerability to addiction and the chemical, behavioral, and social modulators of the addictive process."[42] The board concurs and recommends a research effort led by Public Health Service agencies, including not only NCI, NIDA, the National Heart, Lung, and Blood Institute, and other NIH institutes but also AHCPR, CDC, and FDA.

Federal support for research is needed, even without a settlement. Some research must focus on tobacco-related disease, but the foundation of basic epidemiological, behavioral, social, and biological research is equally important in the long term. Research is thus needed in two areas: (1) tobacco-related diseases and (2) basic underlying factors.

Some research can be driven by a need to fill gaps in knowledge that obstruct specific policy actions. The rates of initiation of tobacco use among youths have risen in recent years, for example, but the reasons are not fully understood, neither are the factors that underlie substantial differences in tobacco use among population subgroups.[43] Smoking plateaued among Caucasian youths from the early 1980s to the early 1990s, but it continued its previous decline among African-American youths, with intermediate declines among Latino youths. Some groups now show an alarming escalation in their level of cigar smoking, whereas use of spit and snuff tobacco has risen among other groups. An understanding of the underlying factors is important in crafting strategies for preventing the initiation and promoting the cessation of tobacco use among the relevant populations.

The section on cessation above indicates the importance of knowledge about what does and does not work. This includes knowledge of basic neuroscience, to discover how nicotine affects cells, as well as knowledge of behavioral and social sciences to understand cessation processes and to study different interventions rigorously. Health services research on the financing, cost-effectiveness, and efficacy of programs with various intensities and costs and on how services are provided in different settings will be as essential to developing better treatments as the discovery of new drugs or clinical trials of drugs and services. Behavioral and social science research is needed to understand factors that contribute to tobacco dependence; experimentation, initiation, and addiction in youths; novel treatment approaches (behavioral and pharmacological) for diverse tobacco-dependent populations; prevention, treatment, and cessation in different age groups; and factors influencing tobacco use and biological differences in health consequences among different ethnic, racial, and geographical population groups.

Beyond the topics directly related to prevention, cessation, and tobacco-related disease, broad basic scientific research is equally important. Some fraction of new funding must support such basic research. The initial findings about health risks came from basic epidemiology, and the current knowledge of nerve cell receptors that guides drug discovery has built on decades of work in molecular and cellular biology. One promising new cessation treatment, the use of the antidepressant drug bupropion,[44] traces its intellectual roots to behavioral knowledge about addiction and drug treatment for depression as much as or more than to studies of nicotine receptors or tobacco use.

California's Proposition 99 set aside 5 percent of its new excise tax revenues to support research. This has produced a research program on tobacco control that can serve as a national model. State research programs are laudable, but research is one area in which federal responsibility is clear. In other areas of biomedical research, federal leadership is unquestioned, and that should also be the case for tobacco-related disease. Public Health Service agencies, including NIH, already have in place effective mechanisms for allocating research funds. The board believes that a significant fraction of the funds generated by tax increases or settlement payments should be devoted to research at NIH, CDC, AHCPR, and FDA as an increment to (not a substitute for) current appropriations.

FDA and NIH should mount research programs to improve future regulation.

Research is needed to inform decisions about regulatory strategy. How to measure nicotine and tar, how to adjust measurements for actual smoking or spit tobacco behavior, whether there is a threshold of addiction, and how tobacco additives enhance nicotine absorption or amplify health hazards are all important questions that current data do not answer. Regulatory decisions about tobacco control, focused on the production, distribution, price, and availability of tobacco products to various categories of customers, especially youths, can build on an existing body of knowledge about regulatory regimes for both licit and illicit products (e.g., alcohol and controlled substances). Some regulatory choices, especially those specific to smoking behavior and nicotine addiction, will require data specific to tobacco. With the prospect of federal regulation, the importance of these data increases. It is by no means premature to start building the necessary scientific and normative foundation for nicotine regulation with the intention of establishing a regulatory framework as knowledge accrues. The board recommends that the federal government create a mechanism to assess current scientific foundations for alternative regulatory strategies and to identify and support areas of research needed to lay the foundation for future regulation. Establishing such a mechanism should be a major priority. It is an essential predicate for the congressional action so strongly desired by the public health community. Moreover, even if the U.S. Congress fails to act, such an assessment will assist FDA with developing and implementing further steps in tobacco regulation under the Food, Drug, and Cosmetics Act. If Congress or the executive branch, as recommended above, establishes a government-wide process, then FDA's process can be a constituent part, and it can focus on the measures over which it has authority. FDA should establish a scientific panel to perform the functions recommended above, even if Congress and other parts of the executive branch fail to do so.

The federal government must support research to clarify the feasibility, risks, and benefits of "harm reduction" strategies.

Health risk is proportional to the degree and duration of exposure to tobacco products. One way to reduce health risk is thus to reduce exposure. A history of product modifications that were marketed as health improvements but did not actually reduce exposure—two examples are filter cigarettes that did not reduce tar or nicotine intake and "low-nicotine" cigarettes that merely led smokers to inhale deeper and longer to achieve the same nicotine dose—has raised doubts about harm reduction strategies, as opposed to complete cessation and primary prevention. The advent of new cessation products, however, has turned attention once again to treating tobacco dependence through long-term nicotine maintenance, to reducing tobacco use without eliminating it, and to designing tobacco products that cause less exposure to toxins. The 1994 IOM report noted great uncertainty surrounding harm reduction strategies, and three years later, that uncertainty is not much diminished. The value of long-term use of nicotine products to enhance cessation is, however, the subject of increased study.[45] In addition, an international body recently concluded that "whereas total cessation remains the ultimate goal of tobacco control policy, reduction of exposure to tobacco toxins should be added to the existing treatment approaches."[46] Many questions can be addressed through empirical research. Can safer tobacco products be developed for those who do not quit? What are their individual and public health impacts? Is it more effective to provide tobacco without nicotine (e.g., nicotine-free cigarettes proposed for marketing in the near future) or nicotine without tobacco (e.g., nicotine gum, patches, nasal sprays, lozenges, and inhalers), or are both useful for different users? How will such products affect nonsmoking teenagers? Would they increase the level of initiation of tobacco use in the short or long term by reducing perceived risk or reduce the level of initiation because such risk is part of the attraction to young people? These and many other questions are closely related to those about long-term regulatory strategies and would rest on some of the same research foundation. That foundation is extremely weak now.

The two principal sources of new public knowledge will be (1) documents made public about studies now available only to private tobacco firms and (2) new research published in the public domain. This implies a need to scrutinize documents that become public in cases such as the Minnesota Medicaid suit to see if information pertinent to harm reduction or other regulatory questions comes to light. More important, the federal government needs to initiate research programs to address the questions that arise in connection with a harm reduction approach.

FACILITATE INTERNATIONAL TOBACCO CONTROL

Only 4–5 percent of the more than 1 billion people who regularly use tobacco live in the United States, whereas nearly three quarters live in developing countries.[47] Economic and political factors combine to make tobacco control efforts less likely and less effective, and a U.S.-centered tobacco control policy will not reach this population. Tobacco will kill approximately 10 million people in developing countries annually by 2030, triple the present mortality rate.[48] Without effective international tobacco control programs, by 2025 the number of smokers will increase 50 percent to a world total of 1.64 billion.[49] Because smoking, along with AIDS, is one of the major growing causes of death worldwide,[50] it is possible to avert the devastating future health toll that these projections imply only if developing countries adopt policies to reduce tobacco exposure and to prevent youths from starting to use tobacco.

Diseases in developing countries are undergoing an epidemiological transition from infectious to chronic diseases. In most developed countries the epidemiological transition has been followed by a behavioral transition to unhealthy behavior, including smoking.[51] In the United States and other developed nations, public health measures are designed to convince people to change their behavior and promote their health. Comprehensive tobacco control policies in other nations, such as Australia and Norway, have clearly reduced the level of tobacco use.[52] One study evaluated the effects of advertising restrictions, warning labels, price, and income on tobacco consumption in 22 member countries of the Organization for Economic Cooperation and Development over 26 years and found that a combination of these measures resulted in decreased tobacco use.[53]

Because the transition to unhealthy behavior has not occurred in some developing countries, these countries have the opportunity to halt the tobacco epidemic before it starts. Yet tobacco control is a low priority in many developing countries, where infectious diseases and other health problems demand more immediate attention. Advocates in developing countries have limited resources to fight government-owned or heavily supported tobacco industries, which bring in significant tax revenues,[54] have a strong lobbying influence, and face few advertising and marketing restrictions.[55]

The international tobacco control community, including 1,800 delegates from 103 countries, addressed the predicted increase in tobacco consumption among women and in developing countries at the Tenth World Conference on Tobacco or Health in Beijing, China, in August 1997. The conference approved a resolution that:

> Recommends governments consider the international implications of tobacco control policies or settlements with the tobacco industry, and to ensure that:
>
> • such measures do not contribute to an increase in the worldwide epidemic of tobacco-related death and disease;
> • the legal rights of those not party to any agreement or policy are fully protected;
> • such measures do not inhibit full public scrutiny on the past, present, and future activities of the tobacco industry; and that
> • the tobacco industry pay the costs of damage caused by tobacco.

The United States bears a particular responsibility in the tobacco control movement because U.S. tobacco companies are major international players, producing nearly 25 percent of the cigarettes in the world export market.[56] The United States cannot solve international tobacco control problems itself, but domestic tobacco policy has unavoidable international implications.

The international market has become more important to tobacco firms: Cigarette exports tripled from 1984 to 1994,[57] and Philip Morris's foreign sales rose from 40 percent in 1990 to 70 percent in 1996.[58] Until recently, U.S. policies generally favored trade export interests over international health. The stark contrast between promoting tobacco control domestically and promoting tobacco exports risks long-term foreign policy repercussions, because foreign nations cannot help but notice the different treatment of domestic and foreign citizens. It can only intensify as the health toll rises in subsequent decades.

The United States must promote, participate in, and contribute funds to the building of a capacity for evaluating and monitoring international tobacco control efforts.

The success of tobacco control efforts in developed countries has largely been due to the cultivation of a receptive social and political climate through the availability of information about the real risks of tobacco use, supported by research on appropriate pricing and regulation.[59] The United States can make a significant contribution to the international tobacco control effort by supporting research on the determinants of tobacco use, including the impact of advertising, promotion, and price; the extent of tobacco-related mortality; the costs of tobacco use; and disclosure of the marketing strategies that induce consumer demand. Although much of the U.S.-based research is relevant across borders, some research must be country or region specific to address the local dynamics of tobacco use. Coordination of international research and program evaluation would provide a thorough, reliable, and accessible information network comprising local studies that follow international standards, along with collaborative overviews from academia and international organizations. U.S. leadership has been powerful in the efforts to combat AIDS; comparable efforts for tobacco control are now warranted.

The board believes that international tobacco control efforts should be significantly expanded both among governments and in collaboration with nongovernmental organizations. Current international monitoring is limited: The World Health Organization (WHO) allocates $60,000 and the equivalent of one full-time position to tobacco control. Special projects, country-specific activities, and additional positions are supported by approximately $500,000 in extra budgetary contributions from a few countries, including $75,000 from the United States.[60] Tobacco-related research has been concentrated in developed countries and receives only $50 per 1990 tobacco-related death ($148 million–$164 million worldwide).[61] Tobacco control is usually best organized at the national level because only national governments can enact most measures. Some functions, however, including monitoring and evaluation, must have an international component. WHO has a program on Tobacco OR Health. Information on that program includes background documents and a series of country summaries. WHO estimates that a strong tobacco control program, with a staff of 150, including a team of experts in trade, national and international law, behavioral sciences, epidemiology, and economics,[62] would demand an annual budget of $150 million.[63] The World Bank has operational policies regarding tobacco use that include recommendations to client nations and has identified tobacco control as a high priority.[64] The World Bank estimates that it would cost $20 million for it to mount an effective tobacco control effort.[65] The International Union Against Cancer sponsors GlobalLink, an international tobacco control digital network. The United States should contribute toward such international efforts. The Koop-Kessler report recommended $150 million in federal funding (or equivalent amounts from settlement payments) for international tobacco control.

The United States can finance the efforts of and provide expertise to countries developing tobacco control programs. Dictating tobacco control policies is both unwise and impractical. The board believes that tobacco control advocates in other countries most often simply need financial and technical support, not U.S. or international initiative, to develop and implement tobacco control programs. A number of international nongovernmental organizations have strong, established tobacco control programs, and the World Health Assembly is drafting an International Framework Convention (IFC) on Tobacco Control.[66] The IFC will move nations toward the implementation of comprehensive tobacco control strategies through a series of individual protocols that will vary in degree to allow a state to be a signatory only to protocols feasible in that country. Through these protocols, the IFC will lead cooperative efforts in research and in program and policy development; share information, technology, and knowledge; meet regularly to facilitate development; address international issues; and finance tobacco control measures. The convention approach is flexible and has proven to be successful in the implementation of environmental policies. Success will depend on several agencies working to support tobacco control, including the U.S. Department of State, the U.S. Agency for International Development, the U.S. Department of Agriculture, and the office of the U.S. Trade Representative.

The August 1997 Beijing World Conference on Tobacco or Health recommended the support, funding, and implementation of the IFC by all governments. The IFC is based on evidence that legislation can lay the foundation for continued research and has the potential to mobilize policymakers in various industries—including agriculture, commerce, and trade, as well as health—to support tobacco control efforts. Individual protocols could be organized by levels of comprehensiveness rather than by subject matter, allowing states to "progress from comprehensive but relatively mild tobacco control measures to a sweeping and complete comprehensive programme of tobacco control."[67] International implementation of the IFC would include the establishment of an international fund to train personnel, fund crop substitution activities, and support monitoring and evaluation of state commitments to international obligations.

The United States should refrain from implementing trade policies that undermine foreign tobacco control efforts.

Section 301 of the 1974 U.S. Trade Act, which "permits the U.S. Trade Representative to investigate and sanction countries whose trade practices are deemed 'unfair' to

U.S. interests,"[68] has been used to facilitate the export of tobacco. When foreign practices merely protect domestic tobacco firms or a state-owned tobacco business, this policy has a reasonable trade rationale, but economic goals must be balanced against the health implications of facilitating entry of the powerful U.S. tobacco industry—with its highly sophisticated marketing and advertising methods—into a new market. A few case studies illustrate how U.S. policies can undermine public health measures abroad.

In Thailand, Section 301 resulted in a compromise between trade and public health interests. Profits from the Thai Tobacco Monopoly made up a significant portion of the government's revenue, and the United States claimed that the introduction of U.S. tobacco companies was solely a trade issue.[69] Thai tobacco control advocates, who had achieved a complete advertising ban in 1988, disagreed, and fought the Section 301 agreement proposed between the Thai Ministry of Finance and the United States. The issue went to the World Trade Organization, and in 1990, a General Agreement on Tariffs and Trade (GATT) panel evaluated Thai restrictions on the imports of and the internal taxes on cigarettes that Thailand maintained were necessary for public health.[70]

GATT found that Thailand could "give priority to human health over trade liberalization" as long as the proposed measure was "necessary."[71] The panel determined that "Thailand's practice of permitting the sale of domestic cigarettes while not permitting the importation of foreign cigarettes was not 'necessary,' "[72] but that requiring foreign tobacco companies to abide by regulations that applied equally to domestic and foreign tobacco products was appropriate. The GATT decision states that restrictions on the advertising, promotion, and sale are allowable "provided they do not thereby accord treatment to imported products less favorable than that accorded to 'like' products of national origin."

In Taiwan, protectionist trade practices limited foreign brands to 1 percent of the market, in part because they sold for triple the price of brands produced by the government monopoly.[73] Comprehensive tobacco control programs were being developed in 1988, however, when the United States used Section 301 to open the market. Taiwan proposed retaining advertising restrictions to prevent foreign tobacco companies from targeting young people, but the United States rejected such restrictions and within two years the smoking rate among high school students increased 50 percent.[74] Concerned Taiwanese health officials tried to limit U.S. promotions, but the United States claimed that the restrictions did not qualify as health measures and again threatened sanctions.[75] Although Taiwan's trade practices were initially discriminatory, the introduction of U.S. tobacco products undermined public health initiatives.

In Japan, Section 301 was used to place U.S. tobacco products on an even footing with domestic ones. Before the United States threatened sanctions against Japan in 1986, the Japanese government encouraged tobacco use and employed discriminatory trade practices. Japanese government policies were aimed not at tobacco control but at expanding and protecting a domestic monopoly. Japan's native tobacco industry, including the government monopoly Japan Tobacco, Inc., was protected. In the face of a 90 percent tariff, foreign brands held only 2 percent of the market.[76] Once the market was opened, U.S. cigarette brands accounted for 95 percent of import sales, and within the first year they captured 10 percent of the total market.[77] Even in Japan, where tobacco control efforts are minimal, the introduction of U.S. cigarettes under Section 301 had the regrettable effect of contributing to an increase in overall tobacco consumption, especially among those under age 20. The trade goal was appropriate given Japan's discriminatory trade practices and lack of antismoking health campaigns, but U.S. action, including active advertising and promotion by the U.S. firms that gained entry through U.S. government efforts, also led to increased consumption, most tellingly among youths.

Adverse health impacts militate against invoking Section 301 to facilitate export of tobacco products. Even when the purpose is solely to open unfair markets in countries that have not undertaken significant measures for tobacco control, such as Japan, the health impact should be taken into account before invoking Section 301. In cases in which national governments are actively attempting to rein in tobacco use, U.S. action to facilitate the entry of U.S. tobacco products is clearly in conflict with the public health policies of the foreign governments and is even less justified.

Most countries with unfair tobacco trade practices also protect other industries whose products do not have the adverse health effects of tobacco products. The U.S. Trade Representative should focus first on those products that confer trade benefits without the dire health consequences of tobacco products. A provision new to the 1998 appropriations act for the U.S. Department of Commerce directs the U.S. Trade Representative to use Section 301 for tobacco products only in very limited circumstances.[78] The current administration has signaled that any tobacco-related dealings of the U.S. Trade Representative will include consultations with the Department of Health and Human Services. U.S. actions that conflict with credible tobacco control efforts in other countries are clearly inappropriate.

The United States can study and learn from effective foreign tobacco control policies.

The United States has the potential to influence international policy significantly. A handful of countries have been in the forefront of tobacco control for decades and are well in advance of the United States. Familiarity with their successes and failures can help predict the efficacy of proposed U.S. tobacco control measures. International data consistently indicate, for example, that in many diverse countries, price increases and bans on advertising and promotion and on smoking in public places reduce consumption.[79] The international expert panel on nicotine maintenance without tobacco, cited above, is another example of how international groups can enhance tobacco control efforts.

The Koop-Kessler Report notes that U.S. leadership in tobacco control is not only a domestic issue but is also a foreign policy issue.[80] U.S. tobacco policy will be an important international benchmark, and it should therefore be a high one. As the home of large, multinational tobacco companies, the United States can set standards for tobacco production and marketing and can "ensure that the conduct of U.S. corporations abroad is consistent with our domestic policies and national values."[81] The Koop-Kessler report recommends several principles for addressing international issues, including promoting the international adoption of U.S. standards, emphasizing public health over trade interests, funding international tobacco control activities, and preventing U.S. tobacco companies from undermining these efforts.[82] It also warns that "a weak scheme of U.S. tobacco control regulation will be cited aggressively by tobacco lobbyists in other countries and international bodies as grounds for resisting stronger regulation."

The United States has a significant self-interest in developing a strong international tobacco control policy. The 1997 IOM report, *America's Vital Interest in Global Health* suggests that by becoming a leader in international health issues, "the United States will fulfill its national responsibility to protect Americans' health, enhance U.S. economic interests, and project U.S. influence internationally."[83]

U.S. government action will often require concerted action with other countries as well. Unilateral actions would merely encourage U.S. firms to shift operations abroad or open the door for foreign firms to take over markets now dominated by U.S. firms, with no change in underlying behavior. The tobacco industry has long operated from an international perspective, and public health measures must be similarly global. Adoption of a comprehensive domestic tobacco control program is of unquestioned importance in the United States, but it will be incomplete without commitment to an international collaborative effort.

SUMMARY

The National Cancer Policy Board chose to issue its first policy statement on tobacco control because tobacco use is the single largest cause of cancer deaths,[84] and because tobacco joins AIDS as one of two major growing health threats worldwide.[85] The board believes that:

• The single most direct and reliable method for reducing consumption is to increase the price of tobacco products, thus encouraging the cessation and reducing the level of initiation of tobacco use.

• Some of the revenues generated should go to support tobacco control measures.

• Lack of a research foundation and incomplete disclosure of proprietary data about nicotine addiction, health effects of additives, and behavioral responses to levels of nicotine and other constituents in tobacco make it difficult to foresee the optimal regulatory strategy. Yet as scientific data accumulate, future regulation of nicotine levels, additives, tar and other tobacco constituents might well be needed. Limiting FDA's authority now is unwise.

• Regardless of whether the U.S. Congress passes legislation similar to that proposed in the settlement, the United States needs a much more robust system for monitoring tobacco use and a stronger infrastructure at the state and local levels. Nongovernment organizations must also be supported, as they hold government and private parties to account.

• Federal research agencies should augment their efforts to gain knowledge about which tobacco control measures are most effective, studied at sufficient dose and duration.

• Research is a federal responsibility and must encompass research on tobacco-related diseases and behaviors, but research to understand underlying factors is also needed. Finally,

• The United States should support international tobacco control efforts and should refrain from implementing policies that would increase the future health toll from tobacco use abroad.

References and Notes

1. Lynch, B.S., and R.J. Bonnie, Eds., Institute of Medicine. *Growing Up Tobacco Free: Preventing Nicotine Addiction in Children and Youths.* Washington, D.C.: National Academy Press, 1994.

2. Centers for Disease Control and Prevention. *Preventing Tobacco Use Among Young People: A Report of the Surgeon General.* Washington, D.C.: Department of Health and Human Services, 1994.

3. Data on youth tobacco use from the University of Michigan's "Monitoring the Future" study (http://www.isr.umich.edu/src/mtf/) (percent respondents):

	1991	1992	1993	1994	1995	1996
Any daily use of cigarettes						
8th grade	7.2	7.0	8.3	8.8	9.3	10.4
10th grade	12.6	12.3	14.2	14.6	16.3	18.3
12th grade	18.5	17.2	19.0	19.4	21.6	22.2
More than 1/2 pack per day						
8th grade	3.1	2.9	3.5	3.6	3.4	4.3
10th grade	6.5	6.0	7.0	7.6	8.3	9.4
12th grade	10.7	10.0	10.9	11.2	12.4	13.0
Smokeless tobacco						
8th grade	1.6	1.8	1.5	1.9	1.2	1.5
10th grade	3.3	3.0	3.3	3.0	2.7	2.2
12th grade		4.3	3.3	3.9	3.6	3.3
30-day prevalence of cigarette use						
12th grade	28.3	27.8	29.9	31.2	33.5	34.0

	Lifetime						Last 30 days					
	1991	1992	1993	1994	1995	1996	1991	1992	1993	1994	1995	1996
Cigarettes, any use												
8th grade	44.0	45.2	45.3	46.1	46.4	49.2	14.3	15.5	16.7	18.6	19.1	21.0
10th grade	55.1	53.5	56.3	56.9	57.6	61.2	20.8	21.5	24.7	25.4	27.9	34.0
12th grade	63.1	61.8	61.9	62.0	64.2	63.5	28.3	27.8	29.9	31.2	33.5	34.0
Smokeless tobacco												
8th grade	22.2	20.7	18.7	19.9	20.0	20.4	6.9	7.0	6.6	7.7	7.1	7.1
10th grade	28.2	26.6	28.1	29.2	27.6	27.4	10.0	9.6	10.4	10.5	9.7	8.6
12th grade		32.4	31.0	30.7	30.9	29.8		11.4	10.7	11.1	12.2	9.8

4. Doll, R., R. Peto, K. Wheatley, R. Gray, and I. Sutherland. Mortality in Relation to Smoking: 40 Years' Observations on Male British Doctors. *British Medical Journal* 309:901–911, 1994.

5. Stellman, S.D., and L. Garfinkel. Proportions of Cancer Deaths Attributable to Cigarette Smoking in Women. *Women's Health* 15:19–28, 1989; Shopland, D.R. Tobacco Use and Its Contribution to Early Cancer Mortality with a Special Emphasis on Cigarette Smoking. *Environmental Health Perspectives* 103(Suppl. 8):131–142, 1995.

6. Lightwood, J.M., and S.A. Glantz. Short-Term Economic and Health Benefits of Smoking Cessation: Myocardial Infarction and Stroke. *Circulation* 96:1089–1096, 1997.

7. Centers for Disease Control and Prevention, Center for Chronic Disease Prevention and Health Promotion, Office on Smoking and Health. *The Health Benefits of Smoking Cessation: A Report of the Surgeon General, 1990*. Atlanta: Centers for Disease Control and Prevention, 1990.

8. Murray, C.J.L., and A.D. Lopez, *The Global Burden of Disease* and *Global Health Statistics,* 1 and 2. Global Burden of Disease series. Cambridge, Mass.: Harvard University Press, 1996.

9. As this report went to press, Senate bills addressing broad tobacco-related issues and introduced since announcement of the June 20, 1997, settlement included:

S. 1060 [http://thomas.loc.gov/cgi-bin/bdquery/z?d105:s.01060:], the Worldwide Tobacco Disclosure Act of 1997, introduced by Senator Lautenberg;

S. 1238 [http://thomas.loc.gov/cgi-bin/bdquery/z?d105:s.01238:], the Tobacco Use by Minors Deterrence Act of 1997, introduced by Senator Smith; the House companion measures are H.R. 2017 [http://thomas.loc.gov/cgi-bin/bdquery/z?d105:h.r.02017:] and 2034 [http://thomas.loc.gov/cgi-bin/bdquery/z?d105:h.r.02034:], introduced by Rep. Bishop;

S. 1310 [http://thomas.loc.gov/cgi-bin/bdquery/z?d105:s.01310:], the Long-Term Economic Assistance for Farmers (LEAF) Act, introduced by Senator Ford;

S. 1313 [http://thomas.loc.gov/cgi-bin/bdquery/z?d105:s.01313:], the Tobacco Transition Act, introduced by Senator Lugar;

S 1343 [http://thomas.loc.gov/cgi-bin/bdquery/z?d105:s.01343:], the Public Health and Education (PHAER) Act, introduced by Senator Lautenberg, with House companion measure H.R. 2764, introduced by Rep. Hansen;

S. 1411 [http://thomas.loc.gov/cgi-bin/bdquery/z?d105:s.01411:], which disallows a federal income tax deduction for payments from any settlement and channels funds to research, introduced by Senator Mack (this is separate from other measures introduced, and passed, to repeal a tax provision of the Balanced Budget Act of 1997);

S. 1414 [http://thomas.loc.gov/cgi-bin/bdquery/z?d105:s.01414:] and S. 1415 [http://thomas.loc.gov/cgi-bin/bdquery/z?d105:s.01415:], the Universal Tobacco Settlement Act, introduced by Senator McCain;

S. 1471 [http://thomas.loc.gov/cgi-bin/bdquery/z?d105:s.01471:], the Treatment of Tobacco Settlement Payments to States as Medicaid Overpayments Prohibition, introduced by Senator Graham, with House companion measure H.R. 2938 [http://thomas.loc.gov/cgi-bin/bdquery/z?d105:h.r.02938:], introduced by Rep. Bilirakis;

S. 1491 [http://thomas.loc.gov/cgi-bin/bdquery/z?d105:s.01491:] and S. 1492 [http://thomas.loc.gov/cgi-bin/bdquery/z?d105:s.01492:], the Healthy and Smoke Free Children Act, introduced by Senator Kennedy; and

S. 1530 [http://thomas.loc.gov/cgi-bin/bdquery/z?d105:s.01530:], the Placing Restraints on Tobacco's Endangerment of Children and Teens (PROTECT) Act, introduced by Senator Hatch.

House bills in addition to the companion measures noted above included:

H.R. 2519 [http://thomas.loc.gov/cgi-bin/bdquery/z?d105:h.r.02519:], the Tobacco-Free Youth Act, introduced by Rep. DeGette;

H.R. 2594 [http://thomas.loc.gov/cgi-bin/bdquery/z?d105:h.r.02594:], the Control Youth Access to Tobacco Act, introduced by Rep. Fox;

H.R. 3027 [http://thomas.loc.gov/cgi-bin/bdquery/z?d105:h.r.03027:] to increase the tobacco excise tax, introduced by Rep. DeLauro;

H.R. 2897 [http://thomas.loc.gov/cgi-bin/bdquery/z?d105:h.r.02897:] to tax tobacco sales through vending machines, introduced by Rep. John Lewis;

H.R. 2740 [http://thomas.loc.gov/cgi-bin/bdquery/z?d105:h.r.02740:] limiting attorneys' fees related to the settlement, introduced by Rep. McInnis; and

H.Con.Res. 184 [http://thomas.loc.gov/cgi-bin/bdquery/z?d105:h.con.res.00184:], a resolution expressing the sense of the Congress that motion pictures should discourage youth smoking, introduced by Rep. Luther.

The board thanks staff of the American Cancer Society and Senate Labor Committee for help preparing this list of pending legislation.

10. Warner, K. University of Michigan. Effects of Price on Consumption of Tobacco Products. Presentation at the National Cancer Policy Board Tobacco Control Workshop, July 15, 1997, Washington, D.C.

11. Denmark, Finland, Iceland, Ireland, New Zealand, Norway, Sweden, and the United Kingdom would all have higher prices even with a $2 increase in the United States. A $2 excise tax increment would produce prices comparable to those in Australia, Hong Kong, and Singapore.

12. Novotny, T.E., and M.B. Siegel. California's Tobacco Control Saga. *Health Affairs* 15 (Spring):58–72 1996; Barinaga, M. UC Objects to Research Restrictions. *Science* 273:178, 1996.

13. Lynch and Bonnie, *op cit.* For more recent figures, see the University of California's Tobacco-Related Diseases Research Program at http://www.ucop.edu/srphome/trdrp/homeback.html.

14. U.S. Public Health Service, *Healthy People 2000: National Health Promotion and Disease Prevention Objectives.* Washington, D.C.: U.S. Department of Health and Human Services (Pub. No. [PHS] 91-50212), 1990.

15. National Cancer Institute Expert Panel. *The Impact of Cigarette Excise Taxes on Smoking Among Children and Adults*, Summary Report of a National Cancer Institute Expert Panel, Cancer Control Science Program, Division of Cancer Prevention and Control, Bethesda, Md., 1993.

16. Warner, K., *op cit.;* also Meier, K.J., and M. J. Licari. The Effect of Cigarette Taxes on Cigarette Consumption, 1955 through 1994. *American Journal of Public Health* 87:1126–1130, 1997; F.J. Chaloupka. The Effects of Prices and Tobacco Control Policies on the Demand for Tobacco Products. Robert Wood Johnson Foundation Conference, *New Partnerships and Paradigms for Tobacco Prevention Research,* Sundance, Utah, May 1997, pp. 213–228; Grossman, M., and F. J. Chaloupka. Cigarette Taxes: The Straw to Break the Camel's Back? *Public Health Reports* 112:290–297, 1997; and Chaloupka, F.J. Testimony before the Senate Judiciary Committee, Subcommittee on Antitrust, Business Rights, and Competition, U.S. Senate, October 29, 1997.

17. Harris, J.E. Economic Analysis of the Proposed Tobacco Settlement. Tab 16 in *An Analysis and Review of the Proposed Tobacco Settlement.* Atlanta: American Cancer Society, 1997.

18. *Impact of the Proposed Resolution on the U.S. Cigarette Industry.* A report prepared for the Conrad Senatorial Task Force, October 8, 1997.

19. Federal Trade Commission. *Evaluation of the Tobacco Industry Analysis Submitted to Congress on October 8, 1997.* Washington, D.C.: Federal Trade Commission, November 10, 1997.

20. American Medical Association. *Analysis, Report, and Recommendations of the American Medical Association Task Force on the Proposed Tobacco Settlement.* Chicago: American Medical Association, 1997.

21. The goal would be payments sufficient to make the brands most attractive to youths less profitable than others. This could be achieved by payments based on youth consumption of specific brands—for example a total penalty estimated to reduce youth consumption to target levels, with payments apportioned among manufacturers according to market share of underage users. The assessments would have to be revised periodically to adjust for brand shifting. A similar effect could be achieved via a tax, although unusual in having manufacturer-specific tax rates. Reassessments could be continued until the goals for reduced youth consumption were achieved.

22. Data were presented by Dileep Bal (California data) and Carolyn Celebucki (Massachusetts data) the National Cancer Policy Board Tobacco Control Workshop, July 15, 1997, Washington, D.C. [see http://www2.nas.edu/cancerbd/ 218a.html].

23. Lynch and Bonnie, *op. cit.*

24. U.S. Public Health Service, *Healthy People 2000, op cit.*

25. Durch, J.S., L.A. Bailey, and M.A. Stoto, Eds., Institute of Medicine. *Improving Health in the Community: A Role for Performance Monitoring.* Washington, D.C.: National Academy Press, 1997.

26. The measure could change without actual behavior change initiation if self-reporting habits change (perhaps due to knowledge that results would be used to raise prices), if the duration covered by the question is not optimal, or if those surveyed subtly change how they interpret the questions.

27. Shopland, D.R. Smoking and Tobacco Control Program, National Cancer Institute, Unpublished data. Preliminary estimate from the 1995–1996 Current Population Survey, October 1997.

28. Agency for Health Care Policy and Research. *Smoking Cessation: Clinical Practice Guideline (Number 18).* Washington, D.C.: U.S. Department of Health and Human Services (Pub. No. [AHCPR] 96-0692), 1996.

29. Lightwood and Glantz, *op cit.*

30. Witsuba, I.I., S. Lam, C. Behrens, et al. Molecular Damage in the Bronchial Epithelium of Current and Former Smokers. *Journal of the National Cancer Institute* 89:1366–1373, 1997.

31. Robert Wood Johnson Foundation. *Call for Proposals: Addressing Tobacco in Managed Care.* Princeton, N.J.: Robert Wood Johnson Foundation, 1997.

32. Pinney, J.M. Review of the Current Status of Smoking Cessation in the USA: Assumptions and Realities. *Tobacco Control* 4:S10–S14, 1995.

33. For details, see the Request for Applications *Prevention and Cessation of Tobacco Use by Children and Youth in the U.S.* at http://www.nih.gov/grants/guide/rfa-files/RFA-CA-98-002.html.

34. Warner, K., J. Slade, and D. Sweanor. The Emerging Market for Long-Term Nicotine Maintenance. *Journal of the American Medical Association* 278:1087–1092, 1997.

35. *Wall Street Journal*, October 1, 1997, p. B12.

36. Centers for Disease Control and Prevention. *Morbidity and Mortality Weekly Report* 46:867–871, 1997.

37. Orleans, C.T. Review of the Current Status of Smoking Cessation in the USA: Progress and Opportunities. *Tobacco Control* 4:S3–S9, 1995.

38. National Heart, Lung, and Blood Institute. *National High Blood Pressure Education Program: 20 Years of Achievement.* Bethesda, Md.: National Institutes of Health, 1992.

39. A query of NIH's Computer Retrieval of Information on Scientific Projects database for 1994, 1995, and 1996 was performed on the terms "tobacco" or "nicotine." The search produced the following counts of extramural awards (grants, contracts, and cooperative agreements):

	1994	1995	1996
National Institute on Drug Abuse	62	54	82
National Cancer Institute	62	62	70
National Center for Research Resources	17	13	14
National Heart, Lung, and Blood Institute	20	8	7
National Institute on Alcohol Abuse and Alcoholism	4	15	12
National Institute on Neurological Disorders and Stroke	9	5	6
Other NIH institutes and centers	27	42	11
Total	201	199	202

40. Cancer Control Review Group. *A New Agenda for Cancer Control Research.* Bethesda, Md.: Board of Scientific Advisors, National Cancer Institute, August 7, 1997.

41. This point is amplified by Stanton Glantz in an editorial to be published in a future issue of *Tobacco Control*, "After ASSIST, What Next? Science." Courtesy of the author.

42. Society for Research on Nicotine and Tobacco. *The Importance of Research in the Development of National Tobacco Control Efforts.* Rockville, Md.: Society for Research on Nicotine and Tobacco, 1997.

43. The findings described below are discussed in several places in Lynch and Bonnie, *op cit.,* especially in Chapters 2 and 9.

44. Hurt, R.D., D.P.L. Sachs, E. D. Glover, et al. A Comparison of Sustained-Release Bupropion and Placebo for Smoking Cessation. *New England Journal of Medicine* 17:1195–1202, 1997.

45. Henningfield, J.E. Nicotine Medications for Smoking Cessation. *New England Journal of Medicine* 333:1196–1203, 1995; Benowitz, N.L. Treating Tobacco Addiction—Nicotine or No Nicotine? *New England Journal of Medicine* 337:1230–1231, 1997; and Warner, K., J. Slade, and D. Sweanor. The Emerging Market for Long-Term Nicotine Maintenance. *Journal of the American Medical Association* 278:1087–1092. 1997.

46. Roundtable on Social and Economic Aspects of Reduction of Tobacco Smoking by Use of Alternative Nicotine Delivery Systems. *Conclusions and Recommendations*. UN Focal Point on Tobacco or Health, Palais des Nations, Geneva, September 1997. Recommendation 6.

47. Jha, P., The World Bank, Washington, D.C. International Implications of the Proposed U.S. Legal Settlement on Tobacco Manufacture, Production, and Marketing. Presentation at the National Cancer Policy Board Tobacco Control Workshop, July 15, 1997, Washington, D.C.

48. Peto, R. Global Tobacco Mortality: Monitoring the Growing Epidemic. Presentation at the Tenth World Conference on Tobacco or Health, Beijing, China, August 24, 1997.

49. Mackay, J. Lessons from the Conference. Presentation at the Tenth World Conference on Tobacco or Health, Beijing, China, August 28, 1997.

50. The World Bank. *Investing in Health, World Development Report*. New York: Oxford University Press, 1993.

51. Koplan, J. Discussion: Developing Countries. Presentation at the Tenth World Conference on Tobacco or Health, Beijing, China, August 25, 1997.

52. Country case studies prepared for the board by Kathleen McCormally provide a snapshot of tobacco control efforts in Australia, Brazil, Canada, China, Norway, Poland, South Africa, and Thailand. These countries were selected to represent different stages of economic development and different levels of tobacco control, as well as for geographical balance; see http://www2.nas.edu/cancerbd/22da.html.

53. Laugeson, M., and Meads, C. Tobacco Advertising Restrictions, Price, Income, and Tobacco Consumption in OECD Countries 1960–86. *British Journal of Addiction* 86:1343–1354, 1990.

54. Prabhat, J. International Implications of the Proposed U.S. Legal Settlement on Tobacco Manufacture, Production,.and Marketing. Presentation at the National Cancer Policy Board Tobacco Control Workshop, July 15, 1997, Washington, D.C.

55. Roemer, R. *Legislative Action to Combat the World Tobacco Epidemic,* 2nd edition. Geneva: World Health Organization, 1993.

56. Yach, D. Settlement in the U.S.A: Benchmark for All or Global Sell Out? Presentation at the Fourth International Conference on Preventive Cardiology, July 2, 1997.

57. Levin, M. Targeting Foreign Smokers. *Los Angeles Times,* November 17, 1994. Pp. A1, A5.

58. Koplan, J. Discussion: Developing Countries. Presentation at the Tenth World Conference on Tobacco or Health, Beijing, China, August 25, 1997.

59. Jha, P. Economic Development and Tobacco Use: The Role of Governments and Developmental Agencies in Global Tobacco Control. Presentation at the Tenth World Conference on Tobacco or Health, Beijing, China, August 25, 1997.

60. Collishaw, N., World Health Organization, personal communication. Tobacco or Health Program, September 15, 1997.

61. World Health Organization. *Investing in Health Research and Development*. Report of the Ad Hoc Committee on Health Research Relating to Future Intervention Options (Document TDR/Gen/96.1). Geneva: World Health Organization, 1996.

62. Yach, D., World Health Organization, personal communication, September 8, 1997.

63. Collishaw, N., personal communication, *op. cit.*

64. The World Bank. *Health, Nutrition and Population: Sector Strategy Program*. Washington, D.C.: The World Bank, 1997.

65. Jha, P., The World Bank, Washington, D.C., personal communication, October 1997.

66. Collishaw, N. An International Framework Convention for Tobacco Control. Presentation at the Tenth World Conference on Tobacco or Health, Beijing, China, August 28, 1997.

67. *Ibid.*

68. Rules, Sanctions, and Enforcement Under Section 301 of the Trade Act of 1974, as Amended, available at: http://www.snado.com/intart1.htm.

69. *Ibid.*

70. Thailand—Restrictions on Importation of and Internal Taxes on Cigarettes. Report of the GATT Panel Adopted on November 7, 1990 (DS10/R-37S/200). World Trade Organization. This report can be downloaded in WordPerfect Version 5 format from the World Trade Organization home page at: http://www.wto.org/wto/dispute/panel.htm.

71. *Ibid,* Section 73.

72. *Ibid,* Section 81.

73. *Ibid,* pp. 711–712.

74. *Ibid.*

75. Frankel, G. Thailand Resists U.S. Brand Assault; Stiff Laws Inspire Other Asians to Curb Smoking. *The Washington Post,* November 18, 1996. P. A1.

76. Kluger, R. *Ashes to Ashes: America's Hundred-Year Cigarette War, the Public Health, and the Unabashed Triumph of Philip Morris.* New York: Vintage Books, 1997, pp. 710–711.

77. *Ibid.*

78. Public Law 105-119, Section 618, states that "None of the funds provided by this Act shall be available to promote the sale or export of tobacco or tobacco products, or to seek the reduction or removal by any foreign country of restrictions on the marketing of tobacco or tobacco products, except for restrictions which are not applied equally to all tobacco or tobacco products of the same type." For the full text, see http://thomas.loc.gov/cgi-bin/bdquery/z?d105:h.r.02267. This provision is associated with the efforts of Rep. Lloyd Doggett, and is often referred to as the "Doggett Amendment."

79. Pierce, J. Progress and Problems in International Public Health Efforts to Reduce Tobacco Usage. *Annual Review of Public Health* 12:383–400, 1991; Roemer, R. *Legislative Action to Combat the World Tobacco Epidemic,* 2nd edition. Geneva: World Health Organization, 1993.

80. Advisory Committee on Tobacco Policy and Public Health. *Final Report.* Washington, D.C.: Science and Public Policy Institute, 1997.

81. *Ibid.*

82. *Ibid.*

83. Institute of Medicine. *America's Vital Interest in Global Health.* Washington, D.C.: National Academy Press, 1997.

84. Shopland, D.R., H.J. Eyre, and T.F. Pechacek. Smoking-Attributable Cancer Mortality in 1991: Is Lung Cancer Now the Leading Cause of Death Among Smokers in the United States? *Journal of the National Cancer Institute* 83:1142–1148, 1991. CDC data on cancer mortality are available on-line at http://www.cdc.gov/nccdphp/osh/mortali.htm.

85. Murray, C.J.L., and A.D. Lopez. Alternative Projections of Mortality and Disability by Cause 1990–2020: Global Burden of Disease Study. *Lancet* 349:1498–1504, 1997; Murray, C.J.L and Lopez. *The Global Burden of Disease* and *Global Health Statistics,* 1 and 2. Global Burden of Disease Series. Cambridge, Mass.: Harvard University Press, 1996.